Dust to Dust

Important Information You'll

Need Once I'm Gone

CHRIS FAIRWEATHER

Note: This document is not designed to take the place of a will.

Published by Berhampore Press
Wellington, New Zealand.

Copyright 2018
BerhamporePress@gmail.com

ISBN-13:
978-1545113554

ISBN-10:
1545113556

Table of Contents

Instructions

This easy-to-complete book is an excellent place to gather useful information your friends and family will need once you've gone.

It provides a place to list information such as bank account numbers, insurance details, regular payments, personal information for funeral planning, and much more.

Make life easier for those you leave behind. They will certainly appreciate it — especially, as in their grief at your passing, they may overlook important things you'd like them to do.

Important Note: This book is not designed to take the place of a will. If you don't already have a *last will and testament* we suggest you get one drawn up as soon as possible. This book is designed to give additional information and clarity to those you leave behind. Having a will is the most important thing you can do to help loved ones left behind, this book comes a close second.

First Things First

Who has possession of your last will and testament?

Name:_____

Address:_____

Phone:_____Email:_____

Name of executor of will:_____

Address: _____

Phone:_____Email:_____

Name of power of attorney: _____

Address: _____

Phone:_____Email:_____

Funeral/Life Insurance Cover Provider (if any):

Name of Company: _____

Address: _____

Phone: _____Email_____

Biographical Information

Personal Information

Date of birth:

Place of birth:

Mother's name:

Father's name:

Sibling's name/s:

Other significant relatives:

Eulogy Help – Highlights of My Life

Early life, schools attended, achievements, marriages etc.

Medical Information

(Handy in case you become infirm)

Doctor's Name:_____

Contact Details: _____

Specialist Name: _____

Contact Details:_____

Medications I'm on:
1.
2.
3.
4.
5.
6
7.
8.
9.
10.

Your views on life support:

Caring for Children and Others Who Depend on Me

NAME	INSTRUCTIONS

Care of My Pets

PET'S NAME	INSTRUCTIONS

Business Interests

BUSINESS	SHARE	ESTIMATED VALUE

Property Holdings

PROPERTY DETAILS	INCOME	VALUE

IF RENTING LIST LANDLORD	CONTACT DETAILS
WHERE IS YOUR LEASE KEPT?	

Insurance Details (house, car, life)

COMPANY	ITEM INSURED	POLICY NUMBER

Bank Account Details

BANK	BRANCH	ACCOUNT NUMBER

Note any automatic payments that will need closing here:

Do not put bank account passwords in this book

Term Deposits & Bonds

DEPOSIT OR BOND	DETAILS	VALUE

Other Investments and Shares

INVESTMENT	DETAILS	ESTIMATED VALUE

Pension Plans & Annuities

SOURCE	DETAILS	MONTHLY INCOME

Credit/Debit Card Information

BANK & BRANCH	CARD TYPE	CARD NUMBER

Debts / Mortgages / Loans

NAME	DETAILS	I OWE	THEY OWE
You can use more than one line if necessary.			

Tax and Social Security Information

Tax Number's:

1. State:

2. Federal:

Social Security Number:

Who Normally Does Your Tax?

Name:_____

Address:_____

Phone:_____Email:_____

Other Tax Information:

Vehicle Details

VEHICLE	PLATE NUMBER	INSTRUCTIONS
Include special instructions about care of vehicles, any hidden keys, and where registration papers are kept etc.		

Donations to Make on My Behalf

NAME OF CHARITY	DONATION
Note: Large donations should be mentioned in your will	

Items of Value & Who Gets What

ITEM	GIVE THIS TO	CONTACT DETAILS

Note on blank page opposite any interesting history of these items.

Items of Value & Who Gets What

ITEM	GIVE THIS TO	CONTACT DETAILS

Items of Value & Who Gets What

ITEM	GIVE THIS TO	CONTACT DETAILS

Clubs, Memberships and Organizations to Notify of My Death

ORGANIZATION	CONTACT NAME	PHONE OR EMAIL

Power, Gas, Phone, and Other Service Providers

COMPANY	ACCOUNT NUMBER	CONTACT DETAILS

Email and Social Media Details

COMPANY	USER NAME	PASSWORD

Facebook: Delete or Memorialize? (please circle one)

Other notes on Social Media:

After My Death

Organ donation?   YES   NO   (please circle one)

Conditions of donation:

_____

Blood type if known: _____

Burial or Cremation?   BURIAL   CREMATION   (please circle one)

OTHER

_____

Please bury me or spread ashes here:

_____

Type of Funeral?   RELIGIOUS   SECULAR   NO FUNERAL
(please circle one)

If religious please specify denomination:

_____

 Hymns/Songs to play at my funeral

1.

2.

3.

Please Invite the Following People to My Funeral

NAME	CONTACT DETAILS

Please Invite the Following People to My Funeral

NAME	CONTACT DETAILS

Please Invite the Following People to My Funeral

NAME	CONTACT DETAILS

Final Letter to My Family

Special Instructions for My Service

Special Message to Mourners

Last Wishes

Words of Wisdom for My Friends and Family

Additional Information for Friends and Family

Remember to keep this book up to date.

If you don't already have a will, you should get one soon.
Why not phone for an appointment with a lawyer now?

Having a will is the most important thing you can do
to help loved ones left behind. This book comes a close second.